Type 2 Diabetes

The 10 Most Important Questions Answered

THE ESSENTIAL DIABETES BOOK

Nhung Nguyen, PhD

ISBN: 1974220427
ISBN-13: 9781974220427

This book was written to help and to inform people around the world about Type 2 Diabetes. This book is easy to read and to consult and will give answers to the most frequently asked questions about diabetes. Hopefully, the science and research works on type 2 diabetes will continue to bring hope to people who are affected by this chronic disease.

Fortunately, even though the prevalence of type 2 diabetes is increasing, it is preventable. Many of the risk factors associated with diabetes are related to lifestyle decisions and can be eliminated or reduced with time and effort.

CONTENTS

ACKNOWLEDGMENTS

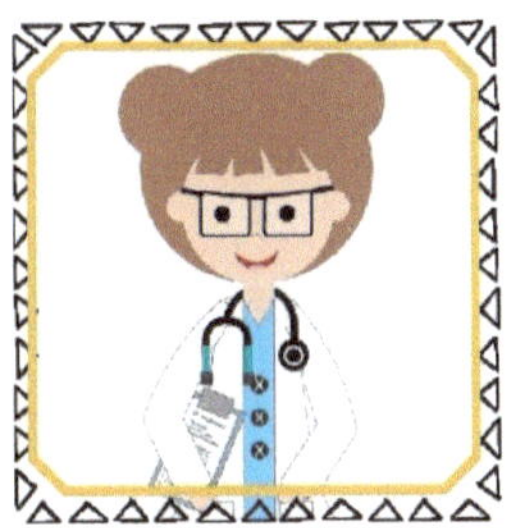

I would like to express my gratitude to the many people who provided support during my studies, research, and projects over the past few years and to all of those who have offered help and who have assisted in the editing, proofreading, and design of this book.

I would like to thank the g.c.e. foundation for encouraging me to publish this book. Above all, I want to thank my daughter, my husband, my family, my friends, my teachers, my team, my partners, and collaborators, who supported and encouraged me in spite of all the time it took me away from them for many years and in order to pursue my researches and projects on diabetes, cholesterol, obesity, and on other chronic diseases. It was a long and difficult journey sometimes but my desire to help people always helped me to go through this process and challenge.

Last and not least: I want to thank all those who have been with me over the course of the years and whose names are not mentioned on this page. Without their love and support, our current research and this book would not have become a reality.

I hope you will enjoy this guide on type 2 diabetes that can be very helpful for people who are affected by this chronic disease and for their friends and family to help them understand it better.

Sincerely,
Nhung Nguyen, PhD

Comments/feedback/media: type2diabetes@mail.com
(Send us a short email and you'll receive a list of the top 10 super foods for diabetes).

Introduction

The International Diabetes Federation reports that more than 380 million people around the world are living with diabetes and that 90% of them suffer from type 2 diabetes. Therefore, diabetes is the biggest epidemic of the 21st century and is on the rise worldwide.

At this time, 8.3% of the United States population has diabetes. This disease results in problems like heart problems and blindness. It also involves great expenses — about $245 billion annually in America.

Despite all the initiatives of diabetes scientists, researchers, and specialists, the situation is getting a lot worse, with more and more people being identified as struggling with diabetes every single year.

Fortunately, even though the prevalence of type 2 diabetes is increasing, this chronic disease is largely preventable. Many of the risk factors associated with it are related to lifestyle decisions and can be eliminated or reduced with time and effort.

As for what causes this disease, it appears that genetics is the most significant contributor. A parent or sibling with diabetes can mean a higher risk for you to also have the condition. In addition, race also appears to be a factor. If you are an American, an African-American, a Pacific Islander, an Asian or a Latino, you are also at a higher risk.

While genetics does play a role in who develops diabetes, another extremely important element is diet. The typical American diet appears to increase your risk of numerous health conditions, including diabetes. In fact, it is unquestionably a significant element in the rise of type 2 diabetes in the USA as well in other nations. Americans tend to consume a lot of fried food, simple sugars, and sweet beverages, but not enough fruits and vegetables. Your body needs nutritious food to combat illness and remain healthy. If you deny your body these nutrients, you will likely get sick.

The third factor is lifestyle. It seems obvious that people are not getting enough workout to remain healthy, considering that over 60% of Americans are overweight or obese. Obesity is a major risk factor when it comes to type 2 diabetes, with 90% of diabetic people being overweight or obese. Frequent exercise is essential to lose weight and to remain healthy.

Note, however, that these are simply factors that make it more likely for you to become diabetic; it does not mean that you will definitely develop the disease.

We will go through these points in detail in the succeeding sections of this book. Other topics that will be covered are the kinds of diabetes, the most crucial signs to look out for, things you can do to diminish the risk of diabetes, and important diabetes management methods.

If you are at risk of developing diabetes or have already been diagnosed with it, use this book to teach yourself further about this dreadful disease and the best lifestyle habits and treatment available for you.

<u>Diabetes: Facts and Figures</u>

Estimated number of people with diabetes worldwide and per region in 2015 and 2040 (20-79 years)

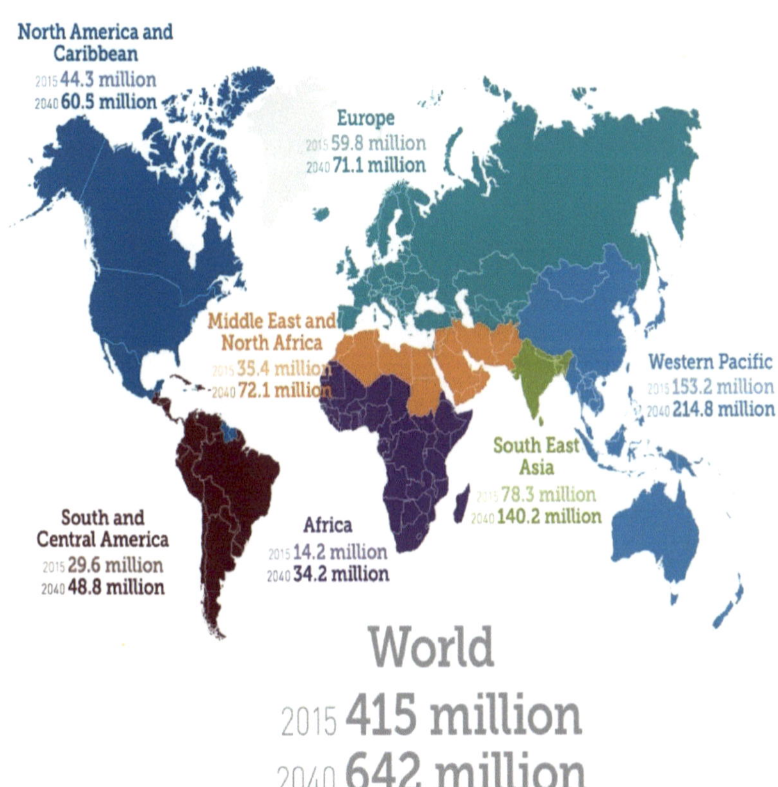

source: www.idf.org

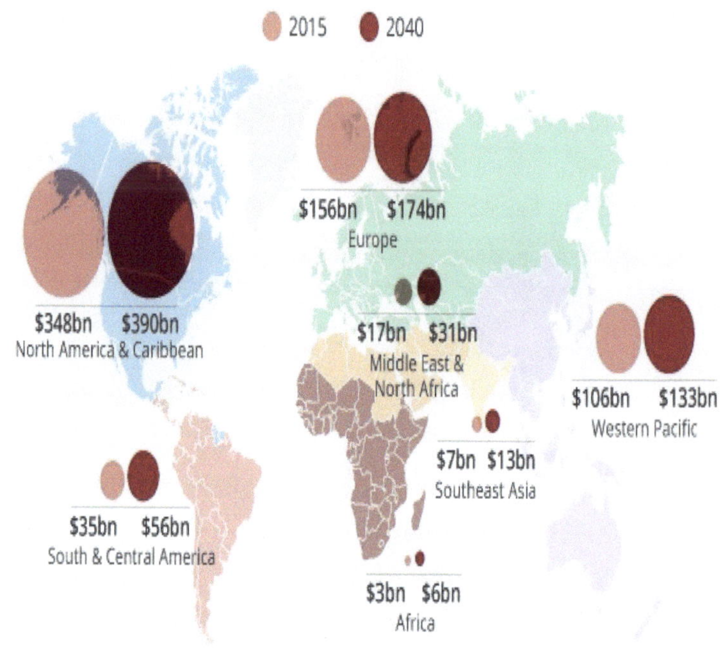

source: www.statista.com

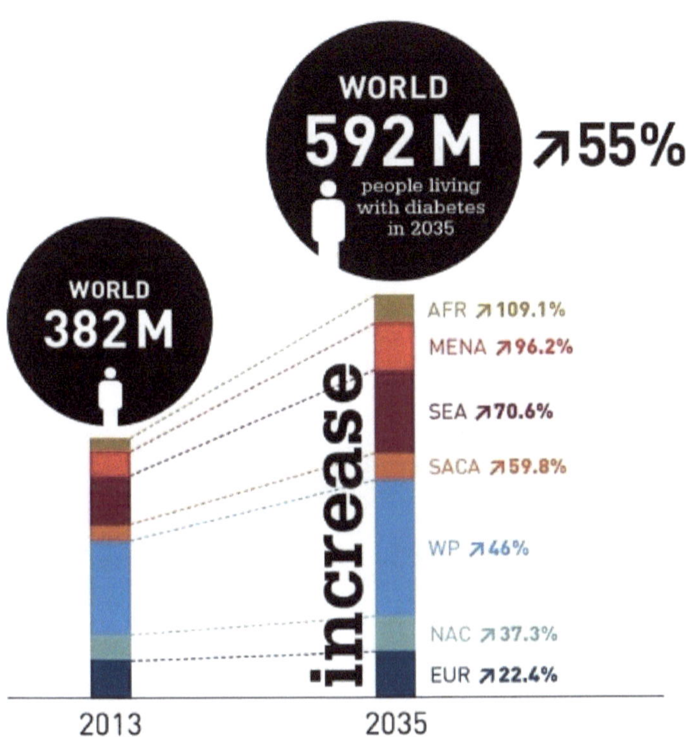

source: www.idf.org

#1 How does type 2 diabetes differ from the other kinds of diabetes?

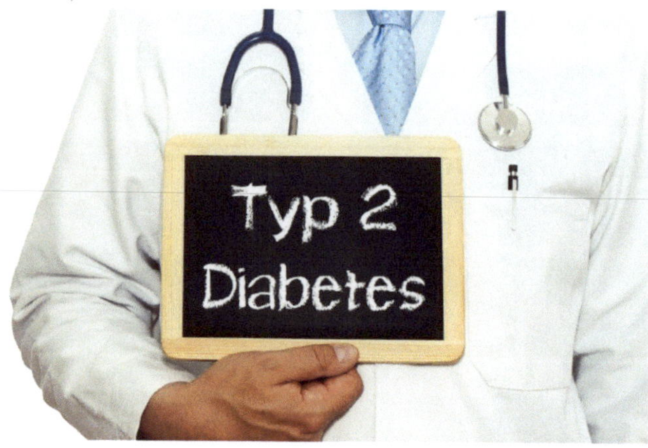

There are several kinds of diabetes, each with its own list of symptoms and causes.

Type 1 Diabetes

Type 1 diabetes can occur at any age, but it is more common among people below 20 years old and is caused by the body's failure to create the insulin needed by the body to function properly. Because of this, type 1 diabetes is also known as insulin-dependent diabetes or juvenile diabetes.

This type of diabetes cannot be prevented as it is caused by a malfunction in an individual's autoimmune reaction. In type 1 diabetes, the pancreas does not produce insulin but it can be managed through insulin treatment and by carefully monitoring blood glucose levels. Type 1 diabetes is much less common than type 2 diabetes and it accounts for 5% - 10% of all diabetes cases.

Type 2 Diabetes

The second — and more common — type of diabetes is type 2 diabetes. In fact, type 2 diabetes is one of the most prevalent illnesses in the USA today. People around the age of 40 and above are often the ones with this kind of diabetes. It is also called "adult-onset" diabetes; however, this term isn't truly accurate nowadays, as some obese teenagers within the USA have also developed this disease. With type 2 diabetes, the body does create insulin but it no longer reacts to it. Because of this, the blood sugar level spikes.

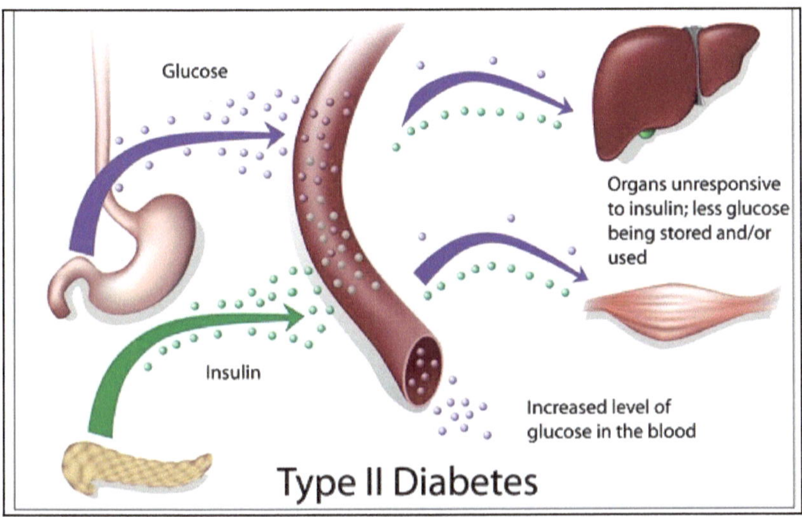

Then there's also one kind of diabetes called gestational diabetes. This type occurs in expectant mothers, usually within the second trimester until the end of pregnancy. Not all pregnant women develop this, however, and the risk is not towards the mom but more towards the developing fetus.

Along with the difference in nature and causes between type 1 and type 2 diabetes, their remedies vary as well. Those struggling with type 1 should provide insulin at frequent times to their systems to manage their blood sugar, but an individual with type 2 may never need to do this. The primary emphases of type 2 remedies are proper diet and correct medication. Nevertheless, an effective diabetes diet may help with type 1 as well.

Individuals with diabetes need to ensure they are consuming a strict diet and looking after their health. Doing some exercises is also important, plus cooperation with their physician (if needed) and obtaining the correct treatment for them. People's bodies vary, so different people may need different kinds of treatment.

#2 Are you at risk of developing type 2 diabetes?

There are many factors that affect your risk of developing diabetes. Though there are certainly a few that cannot be helped, some can be changed. A better understanding of these factors can lower your risk of developing type 2 diabetes and help you remain healthy.

Risk Factors

Bad Diet. Too much sweet and processed foods can increase your risk of developing diabetes.

Being Overweight. Being obese is the biggest risk factor when it comes to diabetes. The body needs to store the surplus calories and fat within the tissues if you are overweight, particularly around the abdominal region. These fatty tissues make the body more resistant to insulin. Fat blocks the insulin, which can trigger diabetes in certain people.

Smoking. Smokers are more likely than non-smokers to develop type 2 diabetes.

Lack of Physical Activity. Physical exercise helps manage your fat by burning calories and using glucose to power the body. This helps your body respond properly to insulin and balances your insulin levels. Exercise is therefore very important.

#3 What is prediabetes?

Prediabetes is a state in which blood sugar levels are higher than normal but not high enough for a formal diagnosis of diabetes. The majority of the people who have prediabetes don't even know they have it because it generally has no signs or symptoms.

Prediabetes raises the risk of developing type 2 diabetes, but there are ways to lower that risk. The risk factors for prediabetes are largely the same as those for type 2 diabetes.

How to diagnose prediabetes

- Prediabetes may be discovered by chance if you undergo a routine blood test or if you go for a routine screening for type 2 diabetes.
- Prediabetes may be discovered if you have risk factors for type 2 diabetes.
- If your doctor orders a screening test for prediabetes (same as the test used to screen for type 2 diabetes).

How to treat prediabetes

Treating prediabetes is possible and reachable and aims to prevent or delay the onset of type 2 diabetes. Losing weight through food and dietary changes and increasing physical activity can highly reduce the risk of developing type 2 diabetes.

Fortunately, it is possible for millions of people with prediabetes to manage their condition and to prevent or to delay type 2 diabetes.

<u>Type 2 Diabetes Risk Test — Are you at Risk?</u>

Check the Bonus section at the end of this book to take the test from the *American Diabetes Association* to see if you are at risk for type 2 diabetes.

<u>Are you diabetic?</u>

Diabetes is simple to test and it only takes a few seconds. The test can be done with your doctor or with a blood glucose meter (a drop of blood is all that's needed).

A normal blood sugar level and the recommended target blood glucose level for type 2 diabetes is up to 6 mmol/l (108 mg/dl) fasting, or up to 8.5 mmol/l after a meal.

A marginally elevated blood sugar level may indicate prediabetes
Above 7.0 mmol/l (126 mg/dl) fasting, or 12.2 mmol/l after a meal, may indicate that you are diabetic.

#4 How can you reduce the risk of having type 2 diabetes?

The fastest way to reduce the risk of having type 2 diabetes (or to reduce the harm it does to your body, if you already have it) is to switch to a healthier lifestyle.

Eat Better

Here are some guidelines you can follow to control your blood sugar levels through diet:

- ✓ Consume more low-starch vegetables like asparagus, broccoli, carrots, celery, and onions.
- ✓ Consume fruits that are low in sugar like kiwi, raspberries, and avocado.
- ✓ Eat more wholegrain foods like beans, peas, and grains.
- ✓ Eat lean protein meals like seafood and poultry. Tofu is also a good source of protein.
- ✓ Avoid consuming food made up of simple sugars, such as desserts, pastries, and soda.

You will find more information on nutrition and diet at question number 7. You can also visit the bonus section of this book to find a list of superfoods for diabetics.

Slim Down

Diabetes experts state that obese people have a significantly higher risk of developing insulin resistance and therefore diabetes. Losing weight can help decrease your risk.

Keep Fit

Several diabetes professionals think that those individuals who have a normal workout plan have a much lower probability of developing diabetes mellitus. Physical exercise helps manage your fat by burning calories and using glucose as power during the workout. The workout makes your body respond properly to insulin and helps balance insulin levels. To reduce your threat of diabetes, try to get at least 15 minutes to half an hour of reasonable-to-high-intensity workout each day of the week.

Stop Drinking and Smoking

Smoking raises your risk of developing diabetes. Drinking is also not safe for individuals who are vulnerable to diabetes. It is not that smoking and alcohol consumption result in diabetes, but they affect the exact same areas of your body as diabetes. *You will find in the bonus section at the end of the book more information about Drinking and Diabetes.*

Get more Sleep

Sleep is very beneficial and can make a difference in your quality of life, as well as the length of your life. It is recommended to get at least 7 hours of sleep per day and to go to bed at around the same time each day so that the mind and the body get used to a predictable bedtime routine.

Some of the great benefits of sleep are that it allows the brain to better process new experiences and knowledge, helps to repair the body, and keeps the heart healthy. Sleep also helps reduce stress and can help improve memory.

Good sleep can also help regulate the hormones that affect and control the appetite, which can have a positive effect on weight management.

Manage your Stress

Stress is one of the biggest challenges people face in our modern life. The ways to relief stress vary for each person but a good stress management includes both awareness of stress and some changes in lifestyle.

Trying to be more in the present moment and not worrying about situations or problems that we can't control may also help to reduce stress. Doing simple breathing exercises can help our mind and body to come back in the present moment. Learning to be more in the present helps keep our mind focused on what we are doing now.

If you feel stressed, try to focus on your in-breath and out-breath for a few minutes.

The key is to learn to recognize the signs of stress in our body and mind and to do simple and relaxing exercises to counteract them actively and positively (yoga, breathing exercises, meditation, exercise, music listening, etc).

We can condition our mind to not stress or worry about things that we can't change or have no control over because there is nothing we can do. We have to avoid, adapt and or accept.

If there is a potential solution to a problem, we should not worry because there is a way to change the situation and we'll work our way through it.

How to relieve stress: Identify the sources of stress in your life, get moving, connect with others, drink water, get enough sleep, do breathing exercises (mindful breathing), and make time for fun and relaxation.

Risk Factors of Type 2 Diabetes

Certain risk factors related to lifestyle choices can increase your risk of developing type 2 diabetes but most of them are modifiable.

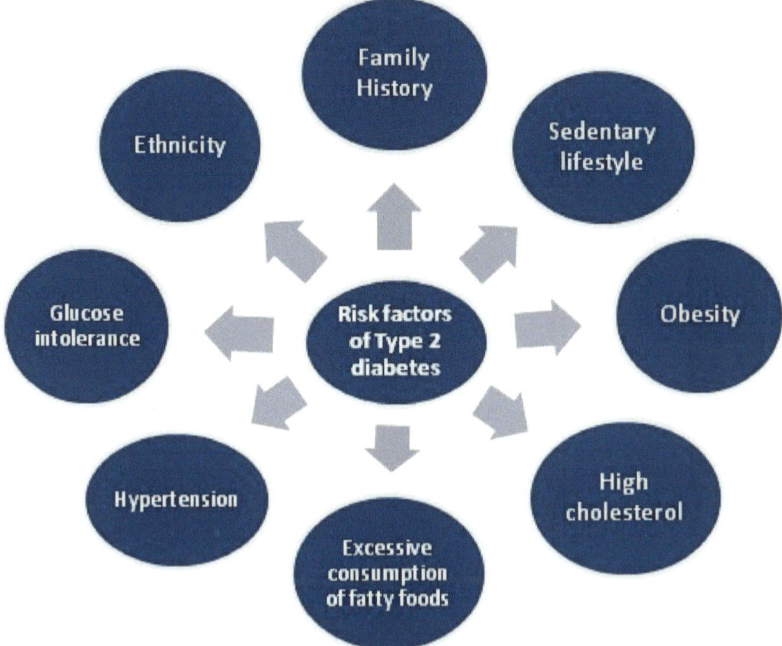

NON-MODIFIABLE RISK FACTORS FOR TYPE 2 DIABETES
- Family history
- Race / Ethnicity
- Age (over 45 years old)

MODIFIABLE RISK FACTORS FOR TYPE 2 DIABETES
- Cigarette smoking
- Being overweight or obese
- Lack of exercise, sedentary lifestyle
- High blood pressure, high fat and/or high cholesterol level
- Poor food habits
- Lack of sleep (insomnia)

People with type 2 diabetes have insulin resistance, which means the body cannot use insulin properly to help the glucose get into the cells. Keeping blood sugar levels under control can help reduce the risk of getting complications from diabetes. The early signs of type 2 diabetes are not always obvious. They can develop slowly over time, making them difficult to identify and many people have no symptoms at all.

#5 What are the warning signs that you have type 2 diabetes?

Indicators of type 2 diabetes should be recognized at the earliest possible moment. This is essential because diabetes is a medical problem but the condition can be handled efficiently at the first stages of the problem, so it is crucial for you to consult a physician when you experience any danger sign of diabetes. The doctor can provide steps that you can take to manage the symptoms of diabetes or avoid diabetic problems.

As we mentioned at the beginning of this book, over 90% of identified cases of diabetes are type 2, where the pancreas creates enough insulin but the tissues of your body become ineffective in making use of that insulin.

Indicators of diabetes are quickly becoming more common while the number of identified diabetics grows daily. The fundamental cause of this increase may be insufficient workout and bad diet. This results in a rise in the number of people who are overweight and who suffer from obesity, which is one of the top causes of type 2 diabetes. Many people with type 2 diabetes watch their intake of carbohydrates and total fat and try to reduce the amount of calories they eat on a daily basis.

Signs and symptoms that can indicate diabetes:

FREQUENT URINATION

High blood sugar leads to increased production of urine and the need to urinate more often. When the glucose level is high, the kidneys react by flushing it out of the blood and into the urine.

UNUSUAL OR INCREASED THIRST

When you have type 2 diabetes, frequent urination due to high blood glucose causes you to lose a lot of fluid and become dehydrated and you will feel thirsty more often.

WEIGHT CHANGE (GAIN OR LOSS)

In people with type 2 diabetes, the cells don't get enough glucose, which may cause the person to lose weight. Also, people who are overweight or obese have more chances of developing type 2 diabetes.

FATIGUE, LACK OF ENERGY, HEADACHES

High blood sugar levels (or low blood sugar levels) can cause extreme fatigue, lack of energy, and even headaches.

BLURRED VISION

Many people with type 2 diabetes may experience blurred vision in the early stages of diabetes or when they start insulin treatment. This blurred vision is caused by fluid seeping into the lens of the eye. It is recommended for adults with type 2 diabetes to get a complete eye exam after they have been diagnosed.

FREQUENT OR RECURRING INFECTIONS

Because bacteria multiply more quickly when blood sugar levels are high, certain infections and sores may take a long time to heal and this could be a sign of type 2 diabetes. Other possible signs include recurring infections, itchy skin, foot problems, and cuts and bruises that are slow to heal.

TINGLING OR NUMBNESS

Diabetic neuropathy can cause tingling or numbness in your feet, toes, fingers and hands and controlling your blood sugar can help prevent it.

INCREASED HUNGER

In people with type 2 diabetes, the insulin level sends signals to the brain that your body is hungry.

SEXUAL DYSFUNCTION

Some estimates suggest that between 35% and 60% of men with diabetes will eventually suffer from erectile dysfunction. For women, statistics show that about 30% of women with diabetes will have some kind of sexual dysfunction.

If you have any of the symptoms above, it is important to contact your doctor or a healthcare specialist. It is also recommended to get yourself checked if you are 40 or older, and even if you don't have symptoms of diabetes (prevention).

#6 What are the lifestyle changes you should do to live without diabetes?

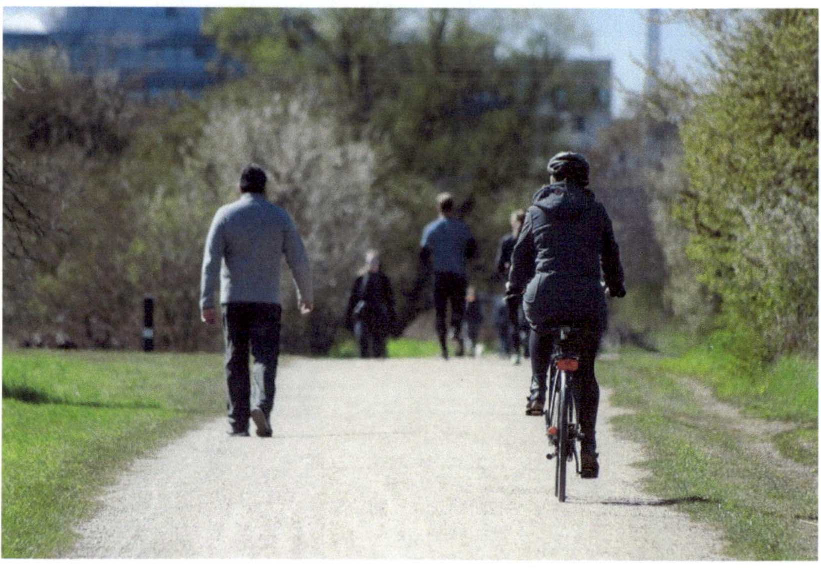

Getting diagnosed with diabetes can be frightening and frustrating. If you do not understand much about the disease, you might even believe that your life is "over," that nothing can ever be the same. Even though it is true that your life will change, you will find diabetic individuals all around the globe who live pleasant, healthy lives every single day.

Simple lifestyle changes

- Get Moving: Walk 15-20 minutes per day.
- Connect with Others: Visit a family member or a friend once a week.
- Drink Well: Try to avoid or reduce alcohol consumption and soft drinks. Drink water, black coffee or green tea.
- Sleep Well: Try to get at least 7 hours of sleep per night.
- Eat Less: Try to cut your total calories intake per day. Eat smaller portions.
- Manage Stress: Try to focus on the present moment and calm your mind with simple breathing exercises or meditation.
- Enjoy Life: Try to make time for fun, activities, and relaxation.

Learn

The key to making positive life changes and understanding diabetes is to know how it affects you. To be able to do this, you have to do your research. Specifically, be sure to find out what kind of diabetes you have, because each kind is managed and treated differently (Type 1 vs Type 2). Understanding your diabetes is the first step to making the right choices when it comes to positive lifestyle changes.

Consult

Some diabetes cases require extremely specific treatment for you to be able to remain healthy and it is important for you to follow what your doctor or health specialist tells you. He will not provide the directions to you until these are necessary, so you cannot "select" which areas of your treatment you want to follow. Be sure to ask if something about your treatment is not clear.

Another method is to examine all of your choices together with your health provider. You might be on a particular plan for treatment, but there might be other options if your current treatment is not working out for you. For instance, if your workout routine is too intense, your doctor can recommend ways to ensure you get the workout you need without overexerting yourself.

Communicate

It is also important to consider that even though you are the one who was diagnosed with diabetes, this disease will influence your loved ones as well. Don't hesitate to share with your family and friends the healthy changes you want to make in your life. It is essential that your family and good friends learn about your situation, what you're doing to handle it, and how they can support. Keep them informed and do not be afraid to ask for help if needed. Your well-being is important, and family and friends can be of great assistance to make sure your wellness is foremost in your thoughts.

Always remember that although type 2 diabetes is a chronic disease, it is one that can be handled effectively. You can still do several, or even all, of the things you want to do (activities, sports, travel, etc). Your illness should not and does not have to control you.

TYPE 2 DIABETES MANAGEMENT

Key elements:

Education: Diabetes education is an important first step and all people with diabetes should be informed about this disease that is affecting more than 300 million people worldwide.

Physical activity: Regular physical activity helps your body control blood glucose levels and is also good for weight loss and reducing stress.

Nutrition: What a person eats plays an important role in regulating blood sugar levels.

Weight management: Maintaining a healthy weight through regular exercise and a good diet plan is important in the management of type 2 diabetes.

Medication: Type 1 diabetes is always treated with insulin but type 2 diabetes is mostly managed through healthy lifestyle habits and may require medications to help in the control of blood glucose.

Lifestyle management: Learning how to relax and how to reduce stress levels can be very beneficial in helping people manage their disease better.

Blood pressure: High blood pressure can lead to different diseases (eyes, heart, kidney, etc) so people with type 2 diabetes should try to maintain a low blood pressure level.

#7 What are the best things to do if you have type 2 diabetes?

Every diabetic remembers when he first starts worrying about diabetes. Being actually diagnosed with the disease is still an overwhelming sensation even when one already suspects that he has it. But finding out that you are type 2 diabetic and have high blood sugar levels does not have to be the end of your world. Therefore, the first thing to do is to stay calm and don't panic. In fact, you can look at it in an optimistic manner. Choose to not just endure. Choose to flourish!

The diagnosis

Just how can anybody not be devastated after being informed that he is diabetic? Although discovering that you are diabetic was not what you were hoping to hear, discovering that you are can result in a happier and wholesome you. This implies that you can now begin to create changes in your lifestyle that will not just enhance your life's quality, but extend it as well. Had you not been diagnosed, you would have been unsure of how close you had been to a wide variety of medical issues.

The first and most typical reaction many people experience is despair. They feel like their life has ended and that they are meant to be "ill" and restricted with their capabilities for the remainder of their existence. But nothing can be farther from reality. Should you accept your diagnosis for what it is — a wake-up call — your life may significantly change...in the best way possible.

Being upset is okay because it provides you with the hostility you will need to fight the illness head on so as long as you use it to create adjustments that are good, your rage can help you. But if you let it result in panic and despair, then you are just hurting yourself. Allowing shame to dominate is not likely to improve your wellness and it is always recommended to try to keep our mind as calm as possible.

What to do

Now, check with your health specialist and if you have diabetes, he will probably suggest that you obtain a blood glucose meter. You will find different types with subtle variations. It does not matter which one you purchase — buy a simple one and use it.

Some aspects of screening are extremely very similar whichever meter you choose. You simply need to understand that you will have an 'ouch' second whenever your skin is punctured. After a few days, however, you will quit fretting about this, as it is more the expectation of pain, rather than the actual pain itself, that affects one the most.

Blood Glucose Meter

Just like how blood sugar meters are available in many sizes, colors, and shapes, so are lancing devices. Plus the lancets are available in different quantities and gauges. The smaller the gauge of the lancet is, the less unpleasant it is to prick the skin. However, if the lancet is fine, you might also find it hard to obtain enough blood needed for the test. And not all lancets are compatible with lancing devices.

Repeatedly using a lancet leads to higher discomfort because the edge dulls and pricking the skin becomes harder. It is also a must to wash both hands with soap and water before screening.

The lancets should be disposed of separately from your normal garbage. You can place them in heavy-duty screw-top plastic containers then seek advice from a clinic, diabetic organization or the local authority on how to get rid of them. The diabetic organization or the local drugstore may have especially designated trashcans for them.

It is also possible to draw blood from other body parts aside from your fingertips. Some kits include accessories to permit this, but this method is less accurate.

Don't Stress

Keep in mind that stress also causes attacks. Attacks that always cause reduced blood sugar levels in many cases are associated with nausea. Meanwhile, attacks that always cause high blood sugar levels are more common and are often related to temperatures. The blood sugar increases simply because there are higher degrees of insulin resistance and stress hormones.

Drink water

Do not forget to consume water. Fatigue can be caused by even moderate dehydration, and consuming coffee, soda, tea, and other caffeinated drinks hinders your rest and can result in restlessness.

Sleep

Sleep is vital as this is when the body repairs itself. Rest and relaxation are also important because they reduce tension and fatigue. In addition, avoid food that makes you feel heavy. Consuming a greasy breakfast can make you feel exhausted, but a low-fat, high-fiber, carbohydrate-centered breakfast will not leave you feeling slow.

Learn about your diabetes

You also have to familiarize yourself with diabetes by learning all you can about it. As you understand it more, you will be guided by your knowledge about:
- What you need to do
- What you need to eat
- Things to avoid
- How to handle your situation

Just then is it possible to start treating the illness to really make a difference.

Eat well

Though a healthier diet is helpful for everybody, if you have diabetes, beginning a healthier diet regimen is absolutely essential to improve your condition and manage the symptoms, especially if coupled with daily workout. Recently diagnosed diabetics are not sure their diet plan can manage their sugar levels and they also fear that this kind of diet regimen is limited and difficult to follow. Don't worry, there are different diet plans that are available and you can still find lots of treats and delicious and healthy foods that you can eat while on the diabetes diet.

Take action

An important step is to apply what you learn because no one else can handle your situation for you. To be able to manage and defeat type 2 diabetes (yes, it is possible), you have to make the effort to conquer it. The earlier you start the options that are good for you, the better your experience will be and the less diabetes will have over you and your lifestyle.

#8 What is the best diet for people with type 2 diabetes?

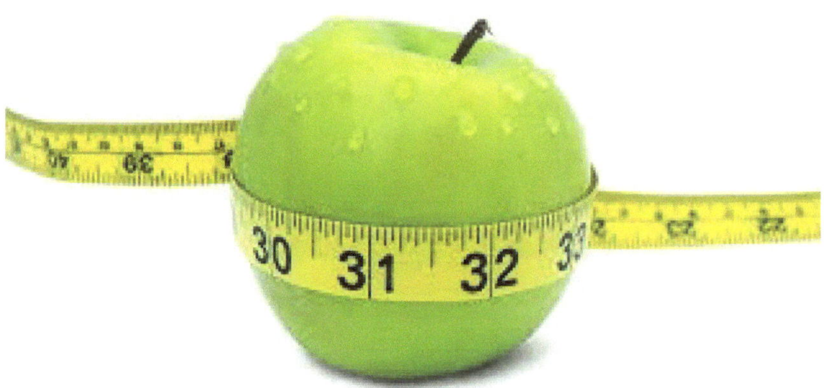

Diabetes is virtually an industry nowadays. In the past, diabetes was just a small problem, something like 1 in about 100,000 deaths. Nowadays, however, the numbers have skyrocketed, that it's actually a worldwide crisis and diabetes is also a big business/industry (with a lot more items available on the market for diabetics every single year).

Well before mass-produced pharmaceutical innovations, people needed to manage their diabetes with diet. Whether it was managed perfectly relied on the person. Fundamentally, each individual has his very own struggle with diabetes and control is crucial if one is to manage it well.

At the moment, there are specific nutritional recommendations produced by The American Diabetes Association for people with diabetes.

Weight control ought to be your primary emphasis if you have type 2 diabetes. If you adhere to a diet regimen consisting of less calories and equivalent levels of carbohydrates and healthier fats instead of specific sugars, you can enhance your blood sugar or body sugar levels.

Food Planning: Diets for diabetes

Undoubtedly, one of the most challenging aspects of managing diabetes is food planning. Consequently and depending on your goals and objectives, it can be possible to work directly with a nutritionist and a physician when you are creating meals intended to preserve normal blood sugar levels. This food program should supply you with the correct number of calories that is required to keep a healthy body weight. *You will also find good information about the best diabetes diets in this book.*

After being diagnosed with diabetes, the sugars in the person's meals should be carefully monitored. You will find two kinds of sugars: simple and complex. A person with diabetes must avoid simple carbs by selecting the healthier substitute — complex carbohydrates. Because the body rapidly breaks down simple carbohydrates, they can result in fast increases in blood sugar levels and so have to be avoided.

On the other hand, the body breaks down complex carbohydrates gradually, which supplies constant power to your body without resulting in an increase in blood sugar. Complex carbohydrates also include fiber that is good for the body. A few examples of simple sugars are snacks, desserts, soda, and fruit juices that have processed sugar. Complex sugars are present in foods like whole grains, greens, and nuts.

Many nutritionists also claim that type 2 diabetics can start to control their body's blood sugar levels by counting carbs. It is recommended that complex carbohydrates be equally divided during the day and equally spread throughout treats and everyday foods. This helps to ensure your body is regularly supplied with fiber, which helps your body to process glucose, enhancing control over blood sugar levels. Fiber can also help by making you feel full longer, lowering the amount of food you eat during the day and therefore reducing weight.

When on a diabetes diet, fat consumption is another thing that needs to be carefully monitored. This is because having diabetes may raise your risk of heart issues such as stroke or coronary attack, which are triggered by large fat consumption that blocks arteries and raises cholesterol. Both fatty foods and trans fats should be reduced when adhering to a diabetes diet. Just stick to food good for diabetics, such as poultry or seafood, and choose lean red meat and reduced-fat milk products.

Many fats also include sugars and so should be included in the daily carbohydrate count to make sure that the body is not getting more sugars than it can handle. By sticking to a low-carbohydrate diet that includes complex sugars, and lowering fat consumption while doing a short workout every day, you can reduce the signs of diabetes and manage your body's blood sugar levels.

Key actions to keep in mind about nutrition:

- Eat your meals and snacks on schedule.
- Choose a variety of foods that are high in nutrition.
- Don't eat too much (eat smaller portions).
- Pick what you like and what you want but read food labels closely.

Best Foods for people with Type 2 Diabetes:

- **Healthy carbohydrates**:
- Vegetables
- Fruits
- Beans (and other legumes)
- Whole grains

Low-starch vegetables: Asparagus, broccoli, cabbage, carrots, cauliflower, celery, cucumbers, mushrooms, onions, green salad, daikon, eggplants, hearts of palm, leeks, mushrooms, peppers, radishes, and tomatoes.

Fruits that are low in sugar: kiwis, raspberries, strawberries, blackberries, cranberries, avocadoes, and olives.

Foods with omega-3 fatty acids (good for the heart): tuna, sardines, salmon, mackerel, halibut, and cod

Healthy oils (monounsaturated and polyunsaturated fats): olive oil, canola oil, peanut oil, almonds, pecans, walnuts, and avocadoes

Although these options for fat are good for you, moderation is key because oil and nuts are high in calories.

Foods to avoid

You should limit or avoid these foods:

Foods heavy in saturated fats, foods heavy in trans fats, beef, processed meats, shellfish, organ meats (such as liver), shortening, baked goods and pastries, processed snacks, sugary drinks and soft drinks, high-fat dairy products, salty foods, and fried foods.

The Most Popular Diets for people with Type 2 Diabetes

Talk to your doctor or to a dietitian about your situation and they will help you to find a diet plan that suits your lifestyle needs and calorie goals. It is also recommended that you talk with a nutritionist if you are thinking of adopting a specific diet, to make sure that it will be suitable for you.

The DASH Diet

The DASH (Dietary Approaches to Stop Hypertension) diet is best known to help in keeping a low blood pressure level and can be an excellent choice for people with diabetes. It is a diet that is rich in fruit, vegetables, and nuts, as well as low-fat dairy, lean meat, fish, poultry, and whole grains. The DASH diet is easy to follow, healthy, and can also be good for weight loss.

The Mediterranean Diet

This diet is very popular and many recipes are available online to help you follow this diet. It is a diet with lots of fresh and seasonal food (fruits and vegetables) and heart-healthy olive oil. A little wine can also be added to this diet.

This diet becomes a style of eating for many people and it can help them with blood sugar control. According to the American Diabetes Association, it is also known to help reduce heart disease risk.

The Vegetarian Diet

A vegetarian diet is made up of foods that come mostly from plants and include vegetables, fruits, and whole grains. A vegetarian diet contains no animal proteins and the most popular vegetarian diet is called Lacto-ovo. It is a vegetarian diet that includes milk, cheese, yogurt, and eggs, but no meat, poultry, seafood or fish. This diet is also good for weight loss but it is important to consume enough protein (vegetal proteins).

List of foods that come mostly from plants: vegetables, fruits, whole grains, legumes, seeds, and nuts.

The different types of vegetarian diets are:
- **vegan:** only includes plant-based foods, no animal proteins or animal by-products such as eggs, milk or honey.
- **lacto-ovo:** includes plant foods, eggs, and some or all dairy products.
- **partial vegetarian:** includes plant foods and may include chicken or fish, dairy products, and eggs. It does not include red meat.

The Part Time Vegan Diet / VB6

The name VB6 stands for "vegan before 6:00 p.m." Therefore, the secret of this diet is to be a part-time vegan. A vegan is a vegetarian who consumes no meat, no eggs, and no animal dairy products.

It is a diet that makes you eat more fiber and less saturated fat and trans fat. This diet also emphasizes being careful about where the small amounts of meat, fish, and dairy you eat are coming from (preferably local, organic and/or grass-fed animals).

The Volumetric Diet

It is a diet that is nutritious and very filling and where you eat a lot of water-rich foods (including fruits, vegetables, and soups). With this diet, whole grains are a staple because they are high in fiber, which helps to keep stable blood sugar levels.

The *Weight Watchers* Diet

This diet is well known in North America and people who follow it have to count "points" instead of calories. Therefore, nothing is off-limits with this diet and you can spend points on anything you want and without having to make only healthy choices. The primary goal of this diet is to help people lose weight but people with type 2 diabetes still have to be careful with how many carbohydrates they are eating in a particular meal.

Intermittent Fasting. 8-16

Intermittent fasting is to make a conscious decision to skip certain meals during the day. It means that the calories are eaten during a specific window of the day and it allows the body to burn food energy. Fasting is free and is available anywhere and is a good method for lowering insulin and decreasing body weight.

The most popular intermittent fasting plans (shorter fasts) are 8 hours of eating per day and 16 hours of fasting. For example, you may eat all your meals between 10:00 am and 6:00 pm. Some people do up to 20 hours of fasting per day and some people prefer to do 24-hour fasts (longer fasts) 2-6 times per month. During the fasting period, you consume no calories but black coffee, calorie-free sweeteners, diet soda, and sugar-free gum are permitted.

When someone is fasting, insulin levels fall and signal the body to start burning stored energy as no more is coming through food. Blood glucose falls, so the body must now pull glucose out of storage to burn for energy.

There are many options that are possible but you should consult your doctor or a nutritionist before starting this diet for short or long term.

Some of the benefits of intermittent fasting:
- Weight and body fat loss
- Lowered blood insulin and sugar levels
- Increased energy
- Improved fat burning
- Lowered blood cholesterol

What type of workout or physical exercise for type 2 diabetics is good?

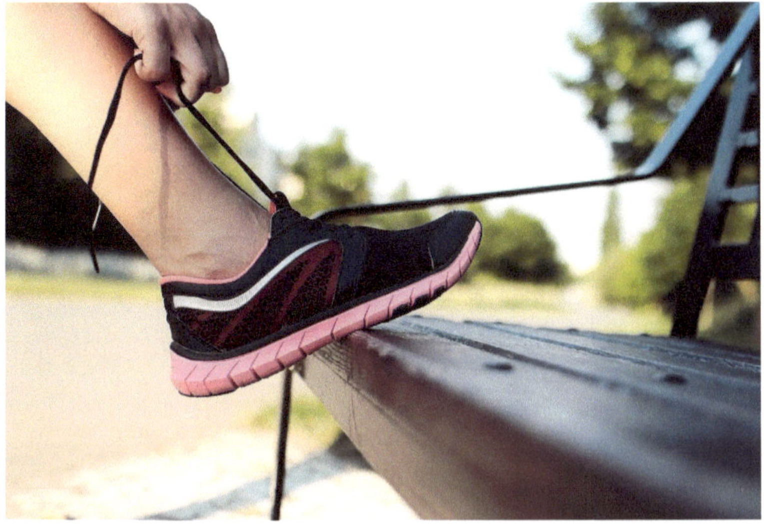

Being active is worthwhile even without diabetes. You will find a number of other advantages of frequent exercise, such as:

- Burning calories — the body proceeds to burn calories at a higher level for some time even after you have completed training
- Helping you manage your weight when you are near your ideal weight
- Helping raise your body's sensitivity to insulin
- Reducing your blood pressure
- Reducing the fat levels of your body
- Reducing the risk of general problems and heart ailments

Exercise can help individuals with diabetes lower their blood sugar levels and control fat. In addition, it prevents heart problems that are typical in those who have diabetes. Workout improves your health and can make you feel happier, healthier, and livelier.

More often than not, it is possible to considerably increase your control of type 2 diabetes with moderate weight reduction, such as 10 pounds, and increased physical activity like walking every day for around 20-30 minutes.

Before beginning, you need to consult with your physician about your intended workout. Your workout routine is determined by whether you have other health issues. Physicians often suggest that you inhale deeper and begin some type of aerobic fitness program that gets your heart pumping. This can be anything as easy as walking but it may also involve cardiovascular dancing, running or other physical activities.

There are several minor risks when beginning a workout program as a diabetic; however, the advantages significantly outweigh the dangers. When they do happen, you simply have to be conscious of them — and be prepared. How the body responds to insulin will be affected by your workout and the exercise may also cause blood sugar to not go too high. Delay before increasing intensity again during these times.

Nevertheless, workout can cause you to feel much better, improve your health in the long term, and reduce additional signs of your diabetic problems. Even though you may have issues whenever you start training, stay glued to your program and look for an answer.

Due to the connection between other health problems and diabetes, enhancing your general wellness with workout and good diet is essential.

According to many studies, being active is among the greatest natural methods to manage your blood sugar levels if you are a type 2 diabetic. If you remain inactive, you will have less chance of managing your blood sugar levels. With frequent exercise, however, you will begin feeling better and your blood sugar levels will be more stable.

There are different kinds of training you can do if you have type 2 diabetes.

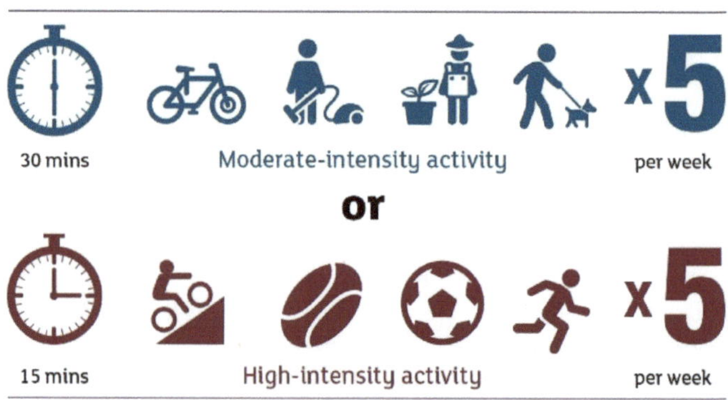

source: www.alzheimersresearchuk.org

High-intensity interval training (HIIT). HIIT is just a type of cardio where you perform hard for a short interval, such as 8–60 seconds, followed by a brief relaxation. It is another type of workout that leads to an amazing afterburn post-exercise and is considered an excellent type of workout if weight reduction is the objective. You can also practice a high-intensity activity for about 15 minutes (five times per week).

Low-to-moderate-intensity cardio. This kind of exercise does not significantly help you shed a massive amount of fat. Nevertheless, it helps reduce the threat of diabetes, cardiovascular disease, and cancer. Furthermore, the lengthier slow cardio you need to do utilizes fat for power (aka burns fat). It, however, generally does not provide you with the greatest benefit for the effort and should therefore be done when you are not doing HIIT or metabolic weight training.

Several examples of a lengthy slow cardio are:
- Enjoying a game in the yard with the children
- Walking your pet daily
- Working in the garden
- Using the stairs rather than the elevator
- Cleaning your vehicle
- Riding your bicycle

Metabolic strength training. This is basically cardio with weights. You can lift a heavy weight for 6–10 reps or a use a lighter weight but perform more reps. In either case, you work hard, burn a lot of calories and fat, and work constantly. The best part is that metabolic strength training causes an intense afterburn, that is, an increased metabolism for 24–36 hours after you stop. Your metabolism is affected by all workout, but it's just high-intensity interval and metabolic strength training that lead to this after burn benefit.

Benefits of Exercise for people with Diabetes

Regular exercise, including walking, can help people with type 2 diabetes lower their blood glucose levels, reduce insulin resistance, boost energy, reduce stress, etc. Doing physical activities also reduces body fat, helps prevent cardiovascular diseases, and helps people with type 2 diabetes to better manage complications that may arise such as high blood pressure and cholesterol.

It is recommended that people with type 2 diabetes get 20 minutes of moderate exercise every day or at least 5 times per week.

If you have diabetes, it is recommended to check your blood sugar level before exercising and especially if you are planning to exercise for more than 30 minutes. An ideal blood sugar reading before exercise should be around 120–180 mg/dL and should be at least 100 mg/dL in order to continue exercising safely. You can keep a nutritious snack (with carbohydrates) and glucose tablets at your disposal in case your blood glucose gets low.

It is also important for people with type 2 diabetes to reduce stress because stress can increase blood pressure and blood sugar levels. There are many exercises and relaxation techniques that can help manage diabetes, such as visualization, meditation, yoga, tai chi, breathing exercises, and more.

Knowing the many benefits of doing physical activity and exercises is the first step. However, you will have to get off the couch and do some efforts in order to integrate some exercises to your lifestyle.

Best tips that will help you to take the next step:

FIND TIME TO EXERCISE

You don't have to exercise for an entire hour to get the benefits of exercise. Even 10 minutes of exercise per day can help. If you are looking to lose weight, short but high-intensity workouts are recommended.

EXERCISING SHOULD NOT BE BORING

It is better to find an activity that you enjoy and you can also ask a friend to join you. If you find it boring to take a daily walk, you can do a dance class, lift weights, etc.

YOU DON'T NEED TO SPEND MONEY

There are many exercises and ways to be active that are free (example: walking, swimming at a public pool, doing squats, etc). You can also create your own little gym at home if you want and this should not cost a lot of money.

THERE ARE EXERCISES AVAILABLE FOR EVERYONE

Even if you are overweight or have limited mobility, there are safe exercises that you can do and that will respect your abilities and your current health condition. Ask your doctor or a specialized trainer if you need more information about the exercises that will suit you best for your specific condition and goals.

#9 How do you select and use diabetes medicines wisely?

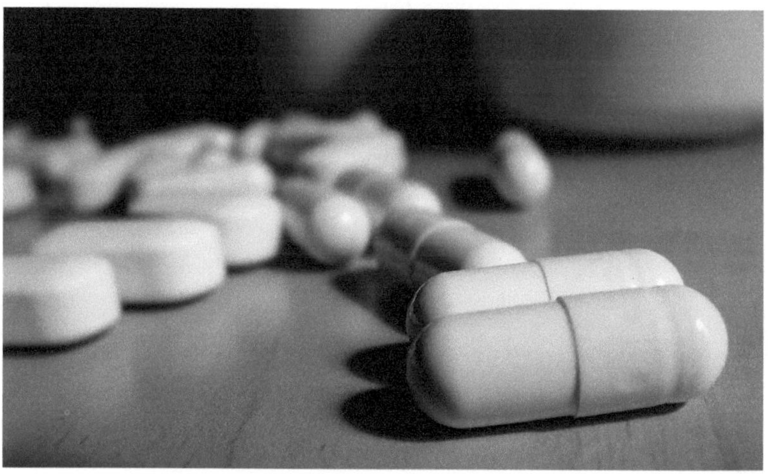

Diabetes is a significant health concern so medical professionals have come up with a large number of methods to treat this illness. Many choices are available when it comes to medication. You will find both natural and prescription medicines. Your doctor will help you select the best medication and treatment for your diabetes. Controlling high blood sugar helps prevent kidney damage, blindness, nerve problems, sexual dysfunction, etc.

If you have type 2 diabetes, you may or may not need medications and insulin to maintain your blood glucose levels and this will be decided by many factors. You should always ask your doctor which medication and which treatment will be most suitable for you and he will consider many factors, such as your family history, health conditions, general eating habits, and blood sugar levels.

All medications are better used with a proper diet plan and combined with regular physical activity.

Side effects may occur while your body adjusts to the medication but you should always inform your doctor or pharmacist if some side effects persist or worsen while taking a medication.

As scientists work to improve the variety of medications to treat type 2 diabetes, other drugs are on the horizon. Researchers across the world are working on new and better ways to treat diabetes and control blood sugar levels.

When changes in diet and increased physical activity are not enough to control blood glucose levels, doctors will prescribe medications. Blood glucose is affected by several organs via several different processes, so controlling blood glucose levels and type 2 diabetes with medication can be a very complex process.

Type 2 Diabetes Medications

There are different types of medications available to treat type 2 diabetes and they are usually organized into different groups to represent the condition that they target.

Examples:
- Increase release of glucose through urination
- Increase insulin sensitivity of liver, fat, and muscle cells
- Stimulate insulin production by the pancreas
- Slow the digestion of carbohydrates

All type 2 diabetes medications have the same goal of controlling blood sugar levels but each medication targets a specific process or organ. When necessary, different medications can be combined to improve results and control of blood sugar levels.

When a patient receives a diagnosis, the most common medication prescribed by doctors is metformin. If after a few months the blood glucose level of the person has not stabilized, a doctor may prescribe a second medication or a different one. If needed, insulin can also be added to the treatment of the patient.

Most popular medications for Type 2 Diabetes

Metformin

Usually the first medication prescribed. It helps your body use insulin more effectively. Some possible side effects are nausea and diarrhea. These generally go away as your body adapts to it.

Pioglitazone

An anti-diabetic drug used along with a proper diet plan and exercise routine to control high blood sugar. It can be used alone or in combination with other medications to control glucose level. Possible side effects that may occur while your body adjusts to the medication are sore throat, muscle pain or weight gain. If any side effects persist or worsen, it is important to notify your doctor.

Sitagliptin

An anti-diabetic drug that helps control blood sugar by increasing insulin release especially after a meal. It can decrease the amount of sugar the liver makes.

Exenatide

An anti-diabetic drug that helps increase insulin release. It also slows down food digestion and decreases the amount of sugar absorbed from food. Possible side effects that may occur as your body adjusts to the medication include nausea, vomiting, diarrhea, and nervousness.

Sulfonylureas

This helps your body secrete more insulin. Some possible side effects are low blood sugar and weight gain.

Meglitinides

These work like sulfonylureas but are faster and their effect is shorter. They can also cause side effects but the risk is lower than other medication.

Thiazolidinediones

These are similar to metformin but are usually not a first choice by doctors due to the risk of heart failure and fractures.

DPP-4 Inhibitors

These help reduce blood sugar levels. They have a modest effect but do not cause weight gain.

GLP-1 Receptor Agonists

Not recommended for use alone. These medications slow digestion and help lower blood sugar levels.

SGLT2 Inhibitors

This is one of the newest drugs on the market for type 2 diabetes. It prevents the kidneys from reabsorbing sugar into the blood and it is excreted in the urine instead. Some possible side effects include urinary infections and increased urination.

Insulin Therapy

Most people with type 1 diabetes must inject insulin but some people with type 2 diabetes may also need insulin. Dosage and number of injections needed depend on each person and your doctor will prescribe what is best for you.

Natural & Organic Medication

Herbs for diabetes are available to people nowadays. Specialists within this area have believed for years that diabetes can be managed with herbal medications. In fact, the effectiveness of those medicines continues to be ranked as amazing. The best part is that these herbs are non-toxic and are effective in fighting off and managing type 2 diabetes. However, it is always recommended to consult your doctor before starting any medication.

Here are a few of the popular natural medications that can handle diabetes efficiently:

Pterocarpus marsupium

This medication is a distinctive mixture of herbs, such as Indian kino, verga, Malabar kino, and Pitasara. It has been used to heal diabetes for several years now.

Bitter melon (Momordia Charantia)

Bitter melon, also called balsam pear, is a plant grown extensively in Asia, South America, and Africa. This folk medicine consists of various substances that are super rich in antibiotic qualities. However, it should not be given to individuals in large amounts.

Gymnema Sylvestre

This plant is effective in assisting the pancreas to produce insulin in case of diabetes. In addition, it boosts the ability of the insulin to lessen blood sugar levels and also reduces the desire for sweets. The plant can be an excellent replacement for medicines that reduce blood sugar levels in diabetics.

Onion

This might be very hard for some to believe, but it is true. Onion substantially reduces blood sugar levels.

#10 What are the possible complications of type 2 diabetes?

Strokes and heart problems are two of the largest killers on the planet. Sadly, when diabetes is allowed to go out of hand, there are many medical problems that can also occur, with heart problems and strokes being some of the most serious. Understanding how they happen and how to avoid them is unquestionably something every diabetic ought to know about.

Exactly why is diabetes strongly linked to heart disease and stroke? Due to some common denominators. Chances are, a person with type 2 diabetes will also be fat or overweight. Carrying around additional weight is hard enough for a non-diabetic, but is a whole lot worse for a diabetic. This extra weight's presence can mean:

- High blood pressure
- Elevated cholesterol levels

Both these conditions are not safe for anybody on their own, but diabetes causes them to worsen.

But, having diabetes doesn't mean that a coronary attack is unavoidable. As we have mentioned in this book, there are steps that you can take to practically get rid of the elevated risk. Nevertheless, the secret is to really apply them.

Diet Plan. It does not mean that you have to give up your preferred meals for the rest of your life. However, it does imply that you have to eat sensibly if you want to reduce your risk for heart disease and diabetes. You can still splurge…as long as you only do it periodically and prepare ahead.

It is undoubtedly much better than increasing your risk, although this may not seem as enjoyable as eating a warm fudge sundae anytime you like.

Workout. We all know how healthy it is to work out but many people still do not take its significance seriously. But think about this: if you did not exercise, what if your physician told you that you might have a stroke or coronary attack? Well, that is precisely what he is saying! You are placing yourself for at least one of those problems to happen. The only question is which one will happen first.

Many individuals suffer not just from diabetes but also from its complications. An earlier diagnosis of diabetes can help an individual stay away from severe illnesses that are related. When diabetes is diagnosed early, it is easier for physicians to monitor the individual's overall health, hence putting any extra medical problems off.

The blood sugar level exceeds the normal range when the pancreas does not function accordingly. Ordinary blood sugar levels ought to be less than 110 mg/dL in the fasting state and less than 140 mg/dL two hours after eating. You can find simple blood sugar level tests that are used to evaluate diabetes.

A person needs to work with his health specialist to stay on the treatment once diagnosed. Remedies may be in the form of shots, diet adjustments or tablets. There are also different kinds of diabetes. If not looked after, all can have harmful results on the body.

It is obvious that the best treatment is to delay the damage by getting meticulous treatment to avoid excessively high glucose levels in the body before it happens. Study has revealed that complications of diabetes — such as vision issues, kidney problems, and coronary attack — can be delayed by sustaining the standard degree of blood sugar below 150-mg/dL, with hemoglobin A1c (HbA1c) level below 7%. The HbA1c test, which indicates your blood sugar level for the previous few months, should be done four times each year to know if your diabetes is properly managed through diet or medication.

Long-term effects of diabetes on the body are often the result of an individual permitting his sugar levels to remain elevated for lengthy periods. That's why early diagnosis is important.

Conclusion

The National Institute of Wellness and Health has been saying for decades that people have been becoming obese. The additional weight that most people are carrying around can lead to severe health issues like cardiovascular disease, cancer, stroke, and diabetes. The number of people with type 2 diabetes is increasing rapidly across the world. Fortunately, there is something that can be done. Some changes in our way of life can help reduce the risk of having diabetes, cholesterol, and other chronic disease and health issues. The most important lessons we should remember in order to live a healthy and happy life with type 2 diabetes are the following:

Eat good food. Eat less.
Move more often. Daily walk or daily workout.
Manage your stress. Mindful breathing.

Cutting off or reducing the signs of diabetes

When it comes to diabetes signs, many people only have to shed about 7–8% of their excess fat to see excellent results. The development of type 2 diabetes slows when you slim down. Your cholesterol levels and blood pressure fall too.

Individuals with type 2 diabetes don't need insulin shots and daily glucose monitoring to handle their disease, but may need medicine to help manage their blood sugar levels. Your primary nutritional objectives are:

- Maintaining blood sugar as steady as you can
- Lowering triglyceride and cholesterol levels
- Lowering and maintaining blood pressure
- Lowering your calorie consumption and doing exercises at least five times per week (15–20 mins per day).

Doctors suggest testing for diabetes at age 30 in people at risk, especially those who are obese or have a family history of diabetes. By implementing a healthy lifestyle routine that is tailored to our needs and schedule, by eating a simple and suitable diet and by managing stress, type 2 diabetes prevention can be done to help us live a longer and healthier life.

Thank you for reading this book!

For comments & feedback: type2diabetes@mail.com
(Send us an email and you'll receive a list of the best 10 superfoods for diabetics).

Bonus: What exactly are healthy lifestyle practices?

Some risk factors for diabetes, like age, race or genetics, cannot be changed, obviously. Nevertheless, various other diabetes risk factors can be changed. The fundamental method to achieve this is by consuming a wholesome diet — not necessarily a complex or super-specialized one — and physical exercise. These easy steps may help avoid diabetes.

Furthermore, if you have high blood pressure or are obese, changing your lifestyle may help stop diabetes. Your well-being treatment company can create certain strategies for you, including diet modifications and workouts that match your requirements. You can also lower your risk if you quit smoking and take some medicines to help you decrease your blood pressure and cholesterol.

Researchers discovered that being obese or overweight may be the single most critical risk element to predict who will likely develop diabetes, based on research recently printed in the New England Journal of Medicine. Research results confirmed, in a 16-year follow up interval, that the enhanced diet (lower in fat and saturated in fiber) along with a daily workout program (at least half an hour each day, five days a week) may considerably help with diabetes prevention.

A medical group called the Diabetes Prevention Study Team mentioned that with enhanced physical exercise program and weight reduction, people at high risk of diabetes can decrease their danger by over 50%. This research was done with over 500 obese people that also had reduced glucose tolerance and diabetes. There are several researches that show that diabetes medicines, training, and healthy eating routines may significantly decrease the threat of developing diabetes. Pharmaceutical labs obviously will not admit that all-natural treatments are cheaper and definitely better. The natural nutrient and nutritional vitamin supplements can help individuals not just avoid developing diabetes but also control diabetes after they have it.

The Diabetes Prevention Plan confirmed that individuals with high risk for developing type 2 diabetes (prediabetes or borderline diabetes) may considerably decrease that danger by using some prescription medications, along with lifestyle and diet modifications. This really is essential, however the above research also confirmed the threat of diabetes may be decreased significantly more through intense lifestyle modifications alone (workout and diet).

The main point here: implementing a healthy lifestyle for diabetes prevention is simple.

Bonus: The role of vitamin supplements

It's both our right and our responsibility to stay healthy. But from outside resources, we need a small aid to cope with our hectic lifestyle and the large and little illnesses around us. Such outside resources include the food and health supplements we decide to consume.

The importance of supplements may seem like an overstatement or an exaggeration but it isn't. Your regular diet barely fulfills our requirements for health vitamins. Besides that, vitamins, herbal medicines, and minerals, if properly obtained, are incredibly inexpensive and mostly safe, without any unwanted side effects. But that's not all. These health supplements do not just help you avoid diabetes but can reverse early diabetes by reducing your insulin resistance and improving your body's function.

There are numerous types of health pills today. Let us take Biocare health capsules for instance. We have a wide selection of them available, with different pills providing different advantages. Let's take a look at some of them.

Adult Vitamin and Mineral Supplements

Multivitamin pills are essential nowadays. These pills meet a few of the deficiencies with the food we consume. These can bring positive effects, regardless of how healthy we feel, because they help our bodies perform effectively and properly. And these multivitamin pills should be taken on the correct schedule to get the desired effect.

Alli-cinn (Freeze-Dried Nutmeg & Dried Garlic)

Garlic is known as a fantastic antibiotic. It is also used to avoid influenza and frequent cold. It is used to address acne and several common illnesses. Nutmeg, on the other hand, is very good for treating diabetes and regulating blood sugar levels. It can reduce the expansion of leukemia cancer tissues and is very successful against arthritis if taken with one tablespoon of honey daily. Nutmeg is just an ordinary food chemical and can increase your intellectual function. Both nutmeg and garlic are also good for people with cholesterol issues.

Bonus: Diabetic retinopathy and bilberries (blueberries)

Diabetic retinopathy is a major cause of blindness worldwide. Bilberries and blueberries may help diabetics avoid it so let us discuss retinopathy and bilberries in detail.

Diabetic retinopathy is a condition that occurs in about 80% of type 2 diabetics after ten years. The Rouget cells that point the blood vessels within the retina towards the back of the eye are damaged by too much blood sugar, causing the blood vessels to develop improperly and leak.

Before the blood vessels are damaged, there's not much harm to vision. The trickle can be fixed by laser photocoagulation surgery but leaves lasting, tiny spots on the individual...and physicians usually "overlook" to alert their patients of the impact.

Bilberries are fruits that are closely related to blueberries but are mostly uncultivated. They are also known in Europe as fraughans, blaeberries, whortleberries, whinberries, winberries, and wimberries.

The orange and crimson substances in bilberries (not to be confused with the orange and crimson substances in blueberries) cannot resuscitate the Rouget cells, however they may stop the arteries from distending, winding, and weakening within the back of the eye. And when small arteries do split, these substances guard the retina itself from death due to air starvation (or oxygen starvation followed closely by unexpected repair of blood circulation).

Bonus: Drinking and Type 2 Diabetes

Can people with Type 2 Diabetes drink Alcohol?

The answer is Yes. People who live with type 2 diabetes are usually able to safely drink alcohol. However, they still need to be mindful of the amount of alcohol they consume to stay safe and healthy.

Most alcoholic drinks contain carbohydrates but wine tends to contain less carbohydrates than popular beers. Beer has a tendency to increase sugar levels and this means that it can have a more important effect on blood sugar levels than wine. Spirits contain a negligible amount of carbohydrates and therefore should not push blood sugar levels. However, if you consume spirits in a special drink, you have to consider the number of carbohydrates contained within the mixer.

Alcohol doesn't have to be avoided if your diabetes is controlled, if you are healthy, and if you know how to manage your blood sugar level.

The 3 Questions to ask yourself before you consider drinking alcohol:

- Is your diabetes under control?
- Do you have any other illnesses that could be made worse by drinking alcohol?
- Do you know how to manage your blood sugar if it dips too low or rises too high?

If your diabetes is not controlled or if you have other illnesses or if you don't know how to control your blood sugar levels, alcohol may cause some significant side effects.

Regular drinking can also interfere with good lifestyle habits that help diabetes self-care. For example, if someone with type 2 diabetes drinks a lot, he is less likely to adhere to good habits and behaviors like doing exercises, not smoking, eating a healthy diet, and taking diabetes medications.

Moderation is always the key when it comes to drinking alcohol.

Therefore, if you are healthy and your doctor doesn't see any reason why you can't drink alcohol, then you should be able to enjoy your favorite alcohol beverage but without any excess.

The liver plays a role in balancing blood sugar levels and it is highly recommended to prepare for it before you have a drink. Therefore, if you have a balanced meal or a nutritious snack before drinking, the food will provide sugar to your body and counteract the effects of the alcohol. On the other hand, if you drink alcohol before you have eaten some food, your blood sugar level will go lower and the liver will be unable to release the necessary glucose into the body to correct it because the main focus will be on clearing out the alcohol.

Aside from eating, there are precautions that people with type 2 diabetes should take to reduce the risk of low blood glucose (hypoglycemia).

5 PRECAUTIONS

- Never be overconfident with your ability to drink alcohol.
- Have a glucometer so you can monitor your blood sugar levels.
- Be sure that people that are with you know how to identify the symptoms of low blood glucose and know what to do if they see them.
- Drink within the recommended limits.
- Drink alcoholic beverages that are low in sugar.

Bonus: Quick Test to see if you are at Risk for Type 2 Diabetes

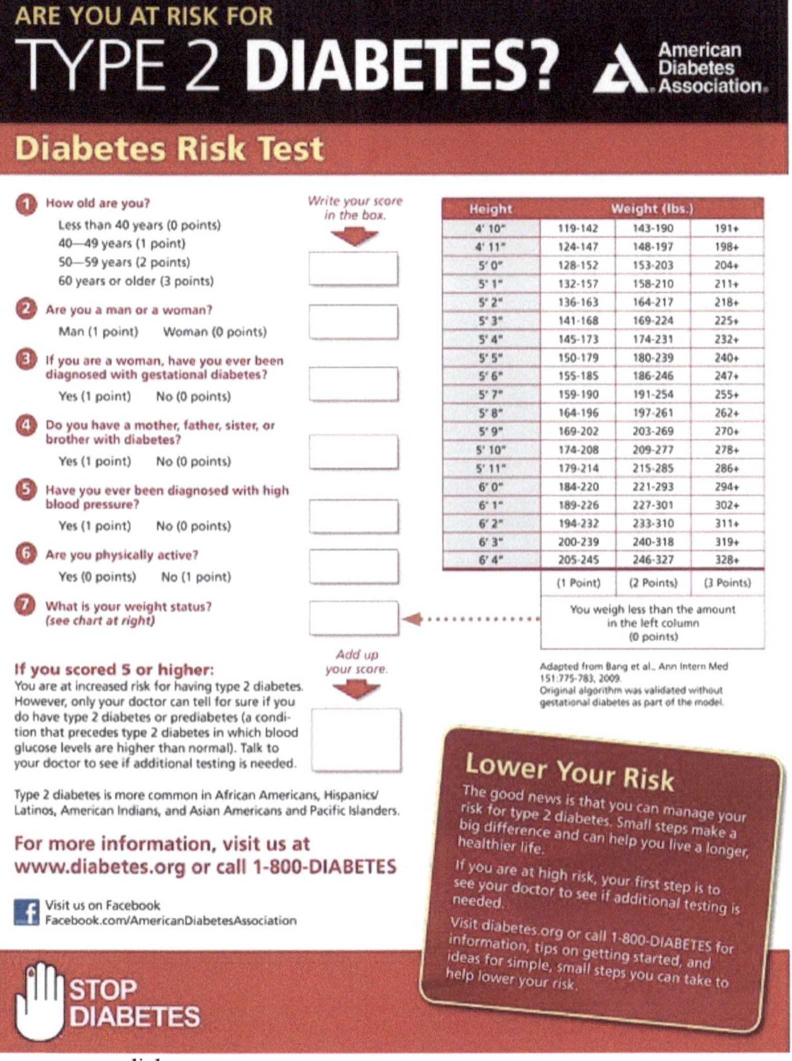

source: www.diabetes.org

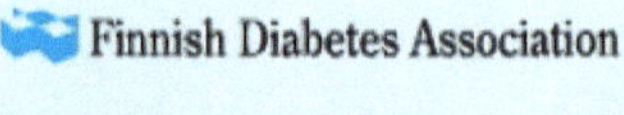

TYPE 2 DIABETES RISK ASSESSMENT FORM

Circle the right alternative and add up your points.

1. Age

0 p.	Under 45 years
2 p.	45–54 years
3 p.	55–64 years
4 p.	Over 64 years

2. Body-mass index
(See reverse of form)

0 p.	Lower than 25 kg/m²
1 p.	25–30 kg/m²
3 p.	Higher than 30 kg/m²

3. Waist circumference measured below the ribs
(usually at the level of the navel)

	MEN	WOMEN
0 p.	Less than 94 cm	Less than 80 cm
3 p.	94–102 cm	80–88 cm
4 p.	More than 102 cm	More than 88 cm

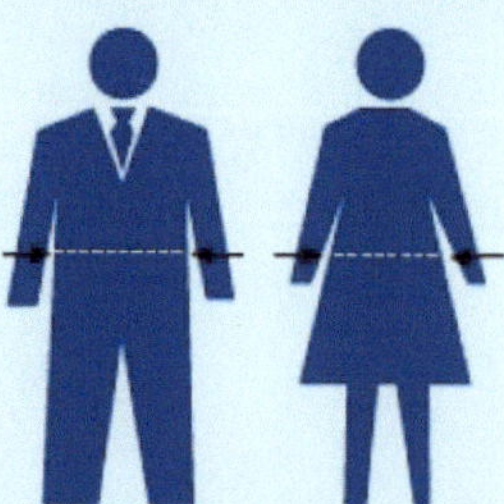

4. Do you usually have daily at least 30 minutes of physical activity at work and/or during leisure time (including normal daily activity)?

0 p.	Yes
2 p.	No

5. How often do you eat vegetables, fruit or berries?

0 p.	Every day
1 p.	Not every day

6. Have you ever taken medication for high blood pressure on regular basis?

0 p.	No
2 p.	Yes

7. Have you ever been found to have high blood glucose (eg in a health examination, during an illness, during pregnancy)?

0 p.	No
5 p.	Yes

8. Have any of the members of your immediate family or other relatives been diagnosed with diabetes (type 1 or type 2)?

0 p.	No
3 p.	Yes: grandparent, aunt, uncle or first cousin (but no own parent, brother, sister or child)
5 p.	Yes: parent, brother, sister or own child

Total Risk Score

The risk of developing type 2 diabetes within 10 years is

Lower than 7	**Low:** estimated 1 in 100 will develop disease
7–11	**Slightly elevated:** estimated 1 in 25 will develop disease
12–14	**Moderate:** estimated 1 in 6 will develop disease
15–20	**High:** estimated 1 in 3 will develop disease
Higher than 20	**Very high:** estimated 1 in 2 will develop disease

Please turn over

Test designed by Professor Jaakko Tuomilehto, Department of Public Health, University of Helsinki, and Jaana Lindström, MFS, National Public Health Institute.

source: www.diabetes.fi

www.ingramcontent.com/pod-product-compliance
Lightning Source LLC
Chambersburg PA
CBHW040229240726
48664CB00001B/67